None for Me, Thanks

*A Journal of Cancer Recovery
with Gratitude and a Feeding Tube*

Robin Hommel

Table of Contents

<u>**Foreword**</u>

I am a cancer survivor. Such an interesting phrase. The word cancer is so ugly, but when you add the word survivor, it becomes hopeful and less frightening.

The thing about oral cancer, my 4 time nemesis over a period of 12 years, is that, especially when caught early, it is rarely fatal. BUT, it tends to recur.

My 4th bout resulted in a more intensive surgery (details included in appendix 4, for those of you who may be interested), affecting my speech and my ability to swallow.

Being unable to eat solid food led me to realize just how food-centric our lives are.

My reasons for writing and publishing this book are:

To share my story
To assist/inspire others on a similar path
To provide resources I did not have, but learned along the way

The title "None for me, thanks" refers to my response the many times I was offered food that I could not swallow.

For those of you new to feeding through a tube; first of all many blessings to you, and I wish you healing and joy. Secondly, please check the appendices at the end for more information which may be helpful in your specific feeding situation.

**Each of us has lived through some devastation, some loneliness,
some weather superstorm or spiritual superstorm.
When we look at each other, we must say, I understand.
I understand how you feel because I have been there myself.
We must support each other because each of us is more alike than we are
unalike.**

Maya Angelou

<u>Chapter 1</u>
December
Weight: 136
Number of medical appointments: 1
(not including hospital stay)

On December 7, my life changed. After an intensive surgery to remove oral cancer, I had another operation to implant a feeding tube called a "peg tube" into my stomach. I was not able to swallow at all, so I needed the tube in order to take in nutrition. My husband and I thought I would have the tube for a few months until I could swallow again, and then life would be back to "normal". We were wrong.

One week later I came home from the hospital – I had been there for 2 weeks. It was a cold and gray day, but to me it was a beautiful day because I was coming home!

A few days after returning home, I had my follow up appointment with the oral surgeon. I found out that, due to the frequency of recent recurrences of cancer, radiation was recommended. Thirty-three treatments, 5 days a week for 6 ½ weeks. We were not completely surprised, but still disappointed to learn about this. Walking back to the parking garage in the rain, I just stopped and sat down on a brick wall and cried.

Because radiation to the head and neck makes swallowing more difficult, I had to keep the feeding tube through the radiation and recovery periods. So ok then, maybe I would get rid of the tube by my birthday in August, and THEN back to normal. Stay tuned!

Our first social outing after returning home was to attend my father-in-law's 90th birthday celebration. I was not able to eat anything at all, but it felt good to join the immediate family and cousins from near and far. One of the cousins, also aged 90, wrote and recited a poem for the birthday guy!

We celebrated Christmas at my sister's house. I was happy to see my family, especially my sons and their families. It was very awkward and isolating to be the only one unable to eat and enjoy the food.

Have you ever thought about the concept of standing out versus blending in? I felt like my inability to eat caused me to stand out in a negative way, when I wanted to blend in. But in other ways, I <u>chose</u> to stand out – friends and family who've seen my fashion choices over the years will back me up on this.

New Year's Eve was the same as any other year. We always stay home and watch movies, and try to stay awake to see the ball drop at midnight. This year I fell asleep early, but the New Year still arrived!

Gratitude for the month:

Extremely thankful for my husband, who took great care of me when I got home from the hospital. Though I felt ok, I needed a lot of help with bandages, gauze, and tube feedings. Thank goodness he is not squeamish at all. I was ready to nominate him for sainthood after all we went through!

Food I miss this month – Reese's peanut butter trees!

**If you can't fly then run,
if you can't run then walk,
if you can't walk then crawl,
but whatever you do
you have to keep moving forward.**

Martin Luther King, Jr.

<u>Chapter 2</u>
January
Weight: 130
Number of medical appointments: 17

Let's take a look at the feeding process using the tube. My peg tube had a plastic disc against my skin, with about 8 inches of tubing on the outside, ending in a cap with a pull tab. To start the feeding, we had to open the cap while squeezing the tube closed like a garden hose, then insert a plastic syringe. The syringe served as a funnel through which we poured the canned liquid. Once we got the hang of it, the process took about 15 minutes. I required 5 cans per day, so at first we did 5 feedings per day. Later we realized I could handle 1 ½ cans in one feeding, so we were able to cut it down to 4 feedings per day. My husband was assisting with every single feeding at first, along with all the bandage maintenance.

If you are new to using a peg tube, here is one tip we learned fairly quickly; keep a towel with you while doing feedings. Sometimes the liquid will bubble right up out of the syringe – we assumed this was caused by gas bubbles. This can get messy, and if you are dressed for work, you'll need to protect your clothes. Keep a close eye on the syringe while feeding and, if the liquid starts moving up, pinch the tube below the syringe. The liquid will eventually settle.

Because at this point I was unable to return to work, my insurance provided some home health care. I had a visiting nurse who came twice a week - she was great and I was always happy to see her. Also, there was one visit from a social worker – the best suggestion from her was to have a "recovery project" – something to keep me occupied while recovering - more on that in chapter 3. An occupational therapist came once or twice as well, mostly working with my forearm range of motion. If you are wondering why my forearm was affected, I direct you to the surgery details in appendix 4.

My inability to swallow meant I had to use a suction machine to remove the saliva. This machine was not easily portable, so I spent a lot of time at home.

While I was at home recovering, visitors were always welcome. My son brought my granddaughter over a few times, and that was the best! My sister and my in-laws visited several times as well. Also, our friend and former coworker visited with her husband. They brought me a magnet with this phrase on it: "Life doesn't have to be perfect to be wonderful". How great is that?

By the 2nd week of the month, I was finally able to DRIVE and to SHOWER! Showering was definitely the priority, but driving was right up there. I had not driven my car for 6 weeks!

My younger son's birthday falls in January. I wasn't ready to head out to a restaurant yet, which would have put my inability to eat on display. Instead, my husband took my son out to dinner to celebrate his turning thirty-one.

There were many medical appointments this month. Radiation consult, CT scan and mask creation, a swallow study, and the radiation dry run. I "passed" the swallow study – no aspiration (no food entering the airway), so it was ok for me to drink liquids and try soft foods such as yogurt. The radiation dry run was somewhat challenging. Wearing the mask as it was attached to the table was difficult, but we muddled through and got it done.

I returned to work (part time) on the 18th. My desk was decorated with streamers and welcome back signs. I had been away for 1 ½ months – my longest stretch of time off work in 24 years!

On the 22nd and 23rd, we had a blizzard! 29.1 inches of snow – it broke the local record for a single storm. Because of the feeding tube, I was restricted from lifting or strenuous work, so I couldn't help clean snow off the cars or sweep/shovel the porch (my usual role in the cleanup). I felt bad watching my husband clearing all the snow and being unable to help at all.

My first radiation appointment was on the 25th. Here is what I later posted on my blog about it:
Picture this:
You are lying supine on a table. A mask over your face and neck connects you to said table. Your mouth is propped open with a hard sponge.
Are you:
A- a character in a horror movie
B- having a nightmare (curse that midnight peanut butter and pickle sandwich)
C- receiving medical treatment

The answer is C! Specifically, radiation treatments for head and neck cancer.
So that is where you will find me each weekday at 3 pm through March 10.

Due to the discomfort of the thickened saliva caused by the radiation, I was unable to continue working. My last day was the 28th.

I read a book on laughter therapy, so we found some funny movies to watch. Some favorites were Penguins of Madagascar and Box Trolls. In addition, I continued a practice I've followed for many years – I severely limit my exposure to the news – it is too depressing. Instead, I seek out websites that share the GOOD news which never makes it to the network news shows.

It became important to put myself in the occasional social situation so I could start getting used to socializing without food. To that end, we went to a friend's birthday party this month. I was starting to feel a bit more comfortable being a non-eater among eaters. The more casual settings, like this one, where people take their plates and sit around anywhere, were easier than "table dinners".

Gratitude for the month:

Thankful for my sons, daughters-in-law, and granddaughter, my husband, snow plows, snow blower, the ability to swallow liquids, my bosses and coworkers.

Food I miss this month – birthday cake!

**Courage doesn't always roar,
sometimes it's the quiet voice at the end of the day whispering
I will try again tomorrow.**

Mary Anne Radmacher

<u>Chapter 3</u>
February
Weight: 128
Number of medical appointments: 22

Three things were at play during the month of February:
Radiation treatments every weekday
Recovery project – blog
Financial concerns and solutions

The actual radiation treatments were quick (5 minutes or less for the most part) and painless. The team at University of Maryland was amazing – patient, compassionate, kind, and funny. We were also fortunate that we only had to drive 25 minutes to get there each day – many people have to travel much farther. The part I struggled with was the feeling that I was unable to swallow with the tongue blade in place. Note – this is not an actual blade, it is a hard sponge on a stick, used to keep the mouth open for the radiation to hit its target. I started taking an anti-anxiety medication, just one dose a day, right before each treatment, to help me relax. I started practicing at home, lying supine on the sofa with the tongue blade in place and setting my timer for 5 minutes. Also helping my attitude adjustment was my husband playing the video for Pharrell Williams' song "Happy" every day in the lobby before they called me in for treatment. I have never tired of that song and will always love it and recall how it helped.

Radiation treatments to this area cause the saliva to become quite thick. It is hard to imagine if you have not experienced it, but I will tell you it is uncomfortable, messy, exhausting to deal with, and just one big hassle. There is also a lot of coughing, and dry mouth. I had to sleep sitting up for several weeks, and sustained sleep was a rare blessing. The good news? It is temporary, and saliva returns to almost 100% normal after recovery from the treatments. There are some beneficial mouth rinses, some homemade and some available by prescription, which are mentioned in the appendices for those of you who may need them.

Having the feeding tube became a blessing at this time. There is no way I could have swallowed food or drink, so the feeding tube = life!

There were some talismans I began taking with me to each treatment. One was a Beanie Baby – remember them? This one was "Peace" bear, a gift from a friend years ago, and he was a good size for me to hold onto like a security blanket. I wore a wristband with the words "Strength and Courage" which was a gift from my son and daughter in law. Pinned to my hospital gown was a "Xena, Warrior Princess" pin, a gift from a friend.

I started the blog on the 6th, and kept it going for 2 years. I really enjoyed writing it, and for me it was a good choice as a recovery project. It gave me something creative to focus on, allowed me

5

to share my story, and gave me the courage to start another blog one day. Here is another selection from my first post:

Here are some things/people I am grateful for throughout this process:
My husband who is with me every day.
All of the technicians who are kind and patient.
The warmed blanket I get when on the table.
My Peace bear beanie baby I squeeze if I feel any stress.
My children and granddaughter (aka Main Motivation) and our families, who have been so supportive.

I wanted to visualize the radiation as the "good guys" beating the cancer "bad guys". For some reason the first good guy who came to mind was Homestar Runner - remember him? I had a giggle in my head picturing an army of Homestar Runners beating up the smaller, weaker army of Strongbads. The next day it was angels vs. devils. Another day I thought maybe a bunch of Dalai Lamas for the good guys but couldn't think who his nemesis would be - all the haters I guess, since he is all love & compassion. I also pictured white hat cowboys vs. black hat cowboys.

I warned the radiation techs that if a spider gets in the room, they are by no means to kill it! I want my chance at getting Spidey sense! I keep saying I'm coming out of this with some kind of superpower.

And just one more – from a later post:

Instead of the good guys vs. bad guys approach, each day while receiving treatment I imagine I am receiving healing and strength. This resonates with me - I always say "I'm a lover, not a fighter!"

Before my surgery, we had thought I would be out of work for a total of about 2 weeks. That estimate turned out to be WAY off. We were not financially prepared for a long absence and lack of paychecks.

My husband runs his own business, so there is no regular paycheck involved. We started to panic once I had used up my vacation time, worrying about keeping the bills paid.

Luckily, family and friends stepped in, and we will be eternally grateful. Along with some financial help from other family members, my son set up a GoFundMe account and got the word out to extended family and friends. What a blessing! We could not believe the amount of money raised; it went well beyond the original goal. We also received a grant from a charitable foundation which helps cancer patients who had been employed in the lawn and garden industry – a friend suggested we apply, and they approved us! I was able to work part time from home, and generally I put in enough hours to at least cover my health insurance premiums. A coworker who lives nearby was gracious enough to carry work back and forth for me. My employer also gave me a payroll advance loan, to be repaid upon my return to full time work.

This experience showed me that I needed to get a better handle on my finances. I was carrying a balance on 2 credit cards. I signed up for a debt management program, which allowed me to save money on payments and have a much lower interest rate on what was a high interest card. I shredded that card and created a plan for getting it paid off within a reasonable time frame.

I continued my laughter therapy, watching more funny movies, our favorite TV show Big Bang Theory, and watching Ellen every weekday. That woman is a blessing to the world, make no mistake about it. Something else to watch if you need a boost – any video by Kid President. Guaranteed to make you smile.

My sister, the best big sister a girl could have, kept sending me gifts. Before my surgery, she gave me a big bag of books and puzzle books and coloring books to pass the recovery time. When I passed the halfway mark in the number of radiation treatments, she brought another gift!

For Valentine's Day, MANY of my coworkers signed kid-sized valentines and sent them all to me along with a small musical stuffed bear. What a nice surprise!

Gratitude for the month:

So thankful for all the financial help from friends, family, and employer. Eternally grateful also for the emotional support from everyone, including my kind and generous coworkers.

Food I miss this month – broccoli!

The greatest wealth is health.

Virgil

<u>Chapter 4</u>
March
Weight: 130
Number of medical appointments: 8

The big event this month was radiation graduation. My last day of treatment was the 10th. They have a big bell in the lobby that is rung by the patient on his or her last day. It was such a good feeling to ring the bell! I also received a diploma.

From mid-February to early April, I was basically housebound other than going to treatments/appointments. I was not driving and was too uncomfortable from the side effects of radiation to get out in the world. One day's big highlight was a walk to the public mailbox on the corner! It was nice to get outside.

My husband's birthday was on the 11th, but I did not feel up to going out to celebrate. My sons and granddaughter came up and took him out to dinner. My family is such a blessing.

Another food event I was sorry to miss in March was brunch with my husband's cousins. It is an annual event and I always enjoyed it, especially the mimosas! Sigh.

One thing I realized while home recovering; there sure are a LOT of food commercials on TV. At first I had to actually look away, because I was so sad I couldn't eat all of the unhealthy junk food they kept showing. Also, a lot of people on Facebook post photos of their dinners, or videos of recipes. It is pretty easy to scroll right by those, so no big deal.

I was not able to visit or assist my elderly mom during this time. I mailed cards to her so she would know I was ok, and thank goodness for my sister, who took care of EVERYTHING Mom needed.

Working part time at home whenever the workload allowed was a big help to me. Spending some time working was a great distraction from my discomfort.

One funny movie we saw this month was *Goosebumps,* starring Jack Black. He is the best

Gratitude for the month:

Thankful for a few 60 degree days, unseasonably warm and pleasant. Thankful for my sister. Thankful for completing radiation treatment.

Food I miss this month – pizza!

For all that has been – thanks.
For all that will be – yes.

Dag Hammarskjold

<u>Chapter 5</u>
April
Weight: 128
Number of medical appointments: 3

Exciting news this month! Come October, I would have a second grandchild! Younger son was becoming a dad for the first time – yippee!

Writing my blog, reading, and coloring – a new-found hobby that I really enjoyed – kept me busy. I had colored pencils, markers (including glitter ones), crayons, and several coloring books.

Finally left the neighborhood and went to Walgreens – woo hoo, an outing!

This month included Passover – I went to Seder with my husband and his family. I had a little matzo ball soup broth.

We went to a friend's birthday celebration at her new home. Great place!

Missed out on seeing another friend who was visiting from California – there was a happy hour celebration but I wasn't up for that yet.

Finally was able to visit my mom – my husband went along.

On the 11th, I went back to work part time. This time I had been out for 2 ½ months! It went very well, so on the 25th I returned full time. There is a small vacant office with a locking door that I used for my lunchtime tube feeding. A little isolating, but I did get a lot of reading done during those lunches!

Because the "tube" part of the apparatus is fairly long, I had to make some wardrobe changes. I started wearing looser, longer shirts so the tube would not be so obviously visible.

My coworker said I should give the tube a name, but I just called it my "alien appendage".

This month saw the beginning of my first pen pal relationship in years - with my husband's cousin. We both enjoyed sending and receiving actual letters by mail.

Gratitude for the month:

So excited and thankful for the new grandchild on the way! Also very grateful to be back at work and in a somewhat normal routine.

Food I miss this month – asparagus!

**Most people ask for happiness on condition.
Happiness can only be felt if you don't set any condition.**

Arthur Rubinstein

<u>Chapter 6</u>
May
Weight: 130
Number of medical appointments: 1

Here is a list of things I will never again take for granted:
Eating and drinking
Having a normal sense of taste
Breathing without assistance
Sleeping lying down
Driving
Showering
Lifting my granddaughter
Running errands

To clarify a few items from this list:

One side effect of the radiation is a change in the way things taste. For a while, even water didn't taste good. To this day it has to be really cold or I cannot drink it. Also, anything the least bit tart tasted SUPER tart. No more Arnold Palmer drinks!

In the hospital in December, I had a tracheostomy (a surgical opening in the trachea to provide an alternate path for breathing and to remove secretions from the airway) and occasional supplemental oxygen.

Another side effect of the radiation was a night-time cough, which forced me to sleep sitting up for several weeks. It sure felt great once I could sleep lying down again.

While I had the feeding tube, I was not supposed to lift anything over ten pounds. Eventually I tested it, and found I was able to lift my toddler granddaughter, though I was still cautious and careful.

One day at work I was in my little "feeding room" and when I tried pouring the liquid into the syringe, it would not go in, and the area around the tube was getting wet. I had no idea what was going on, so I called my husband and he came to help. He tried pouring, with the same result. I was in tears at this point. We called the doctor who had implanted the tube – she had no suggestions (!), so we ended up going to the emergency room. End result? No big deal – the tube had to be replaced – the balloon inside had deflated so it was no longer functional. Apparently the peg tubes need to be replaced every 6 – 12 months! NO ONE EVER TOLD US ABOUT THIS. Of course, when I first got the tube, I would not have thought I would have it long enough to need a replacement! This was just one example of the information we did not have about feeding tubes, and my main reason for wanting to write this book, with the hope of helping other patients.

Another problem we had – listen up, peg tube brothers and sisters – was that the gauze we kept around the tube started sticking to a piece of hypergranulation tissue near the incision (this tissue is a normal development with peg tubes). This resulted in a minor meltdown every night when my husband helped me remove the gauze before my shower. This went on for many days, then my husband had a "Eureka!" moment, and he enlarged the hole in the center of the gauze so it wouldn't touch the tissue – genius! Problem solved; no more meltdowns. If you are a peg tube user, again, please check out appendix 1 – there are notes on the gauze and tapes we used –that was a learning process as well!

I was starting to think I would never end up swallowing food again, but after another swallow study, I was referred to a gastroenterologist to see if my esophagus needed stretching. Another side effect of radiation is a stricture, or narrowing, of the esophagus. This gave me hope! Maybe once the esophagus was opened up, I would be able to swallow food!

This month my sleep improved. For a while I could only sleep for 2 hours max at a time, due to all the coughing. Many things became much easier with enough sleep. I was prone to daily crying over one minor incident or another while sleep was so elusive. Later I found that more sleep = less crying!

Keeping the laughter therapy going, we watched several old Don Knotts movies - laughs aplenty.

Gratitude for the month:

Thankful for spring weather – warmer temperatures made everything more tolerable - and being back in the routine of work.

Food I miss this month – veggie quesadilla!

Energy and persistence conquer all things.

Benjamin Franklin

<u>Chapter 7</u>
June
Weight: 127
Number of medical appointments: 8

This month did not begin well. I had stomach problems and could not keep food down. For a week I did not get much nutrition in at all. After an emergency room trip and an appointment with my gastroenterologist, I got some medicine that helped. We learned that my stomach was not emptying properly. The medicine helped and I was able to eat again. After a couple of months, I was able to stop the medicine and have not had the problem again since, thank goodness.

This is a good point in the story to talk about health insurance and the seemingly random things it covered or did not cover. The expensive medicine that helped my stomach to empty was not covered. I filed an appeal and they finally approved it, but by that time I didn't need it anymore. I was reimbursed for the previous bottles, so that was good – but the process of appealing seemed an unnecessary headache.

Later, when my employer changed health insurance carriers, the new carrier did not cover my canned liquid food. The old carrier covered it 100%. I appealed, still no go. Here is the real kicker – the new carrier covered a replacement feeding tube 100%, but not the food required to use with said tube. Does that make sense to anyone? It didn't to me. This kind of struggle both exhausted and exasperated me.

Once I felt better and got some nutrition in again, I was able to attend my sister's 80th birthday celebration. I tried the sweetest wine they had, but it just tasted like "burning". Alcohol did not work for me anymore – the taste buds did not like it. There was soup with dinner, so I had some of that. I was glad to be there, and I was starting to get used to being at a "food event" without eating much.

I had several sessions of swallow therapy. There was a machine which stimulated the neck muscles involved in swallowing. Sensors were taped to my neck and a mild electrical current passed through, and I drank water and kept swallowing and working the muscles. Then there was a device which measured my tongue strength. There was a tube with a small balloon that I had to press up with my tongue against the roof of my mouth and the amount of pressure was measured in numbers so I had to keep striving for a higher number. I was given a Therabite tool to help increase my jaw opening, and tongue depressors for tongue exercises. I believe the therapy was worthwhile, but it did not correct my inability to swallow solid food.

Gratitude for the month:

Thankful to be feeling better and getting nutrition in. Grateful for the library and for my husband who picked up and dropped off books for me.

Food I miss this month – tacos!

12

Art enables us to find ourselves and lose ourselves at the same time.

Thomas Merton

<u>Chapter 8</u>
July
Weight: 124
Number of medical appointments: 2

I had to weigh myself weekly and keep track, to make sure I maintained and didn't lose too much. Such a strange situation, after several years of Weight Watchers and fighting to keep the weight off!

There were several food events this month. I went to a restaurant to watch my son play guitar and sing. I sat at the bar since I would not be eating, and drank an iced tea. Later in the month I went to a local arts festival with a friend. There were a lot of food vendors there, but plenty of art to keep me occupied – we had fun. Another day I met my former boss at a Starbucks – easy enough to just have a drink there. Also there was a "ladies' night" happy hour with several friends. The only hard part was finding a place to put all of my used napkins – due to saliva issues and incomplete swallowing, I use a lot of napkins. I've since learned to bring a pretty tote bag with a plastic grocery bag inside, so I can contain them out of sight under the table.

This summer, I had several friends recovering from either surgery or illness. Remembering how much it meant to receive a card or some thoughtful gesture as I was recovering, I started assembling and mailing out "recovery kits". Most kits included a card, a coloring book and pencils or markers, a puzzle book, and sometimes a toy like the foam finger flyer rocket – those were a big hit! I bought most of the supplies from the dollar store, so I didn't spend a lot, but I had fun assembling them and the recipients enjoyed them.

Gratitude for the month:

Thankful for friends and art!

Food I miss this month – falafel!

**The great essentials to happiness in this life are something to do,
something to love, and something to hope for.**

Joseph Addison

<u>Chapter 9</u>
August
Weight: 125
Number of medical appointments: 4

I had my first esophagus dilation this month. The opening was only pinhole-sized before stretching! The doctor got it opened up to 6 millimeters. A healthy, un-strictured esophagus opening is 2 centimeters. They can only stretch it so far at a time safely, so I would need to have it done again.

I was not able to swallow any type of pill. Think about that for a moment. Do you take a multivitamin? Supplements? The occasional NSAID for pain? None of those were possible for me. Many meds do come in liquid form, but boy, do they taste awful! My naturopathic doctor recommended a liquid multivitamin. I tried drinking it but the taste was SO BAD (like, green Nyquil bad) – to my impaired taste buds at least. I was able to put it in the tube, so at least I felt like I could get some extra vitamins in. Later I tried a different brand and flavor, but that one also tasted too awful to drink.

We went on vacation, an annual trip to a New Jersey beach town with my husband's extended family. Packing was harder this year, as we had to lug along cans of my food, feeding tube supplies, medications, mouth rinses, fluoride trays for my teeth, etc. (More info on fluoride trays in appendix 1.) It was great seeing all the family, and of course the ocean! We made our traditional jaunt to a favorite seafood restaurant. I was able to eat some lobster bisque broth. Another vacation tradition is eating breakfast out. I discovered hot chocolate with whipped cream was still quite tasty, so that became my standard for breakfast outings.

As a substitute for the food I couldn't eat, I was buying a lot of clothes and books. I've always been a bibliophile, and have created my wardrobe from thrift stores for years, but I found myself buying more than usual. I had 2 plastic milk crates full of books waiting to be read. The clothes were not overflowing my closet yet, so I guess I was doing ok there.

So much for the goal of being able to eat and lose the feeding tube by my birthday this month. Next goal is Thanksgiving!

For my birthday, my older son surprised me by bringing flowers and a card to my work, and then my in-laws invited us over for dinner. For dessert they got an ice cream cake that was all ice cream! No crunchy middle part. I had no idea this type of cake was possible. I was able to eat some!

We decided to go bowling on my actual birthday. It was big fun, with no food involved – perfect! I need to seek out more activities like this – so many social activities revolve around food or drinks.

My younger son and his girlfriend bought a house and we helped them move in at the end of this month! So happy they found a place before the baby arrives.

Gratitude for the month:

Thankful for family, books, air conditioning, and a new house for the new baby!

Food I miss this month – red bell peppers!

**Acknowledging the good that you already have in your life
is the foundation for all abundance.**

Eckhart Tolle

<u>Chapter 10</u>
September
Weight: 124
Number of medical appointments: 4

Our favorite local restaurant had a fundraiser for a nearby town's flood relief and recovery. We bought t-shirts and raffle tickets and drinks. I was wishing I could order a full meal, as a portion of the food sales was being donated to the cause, but we did what we could. It was fun to get out and about.

This month, for the first time in quite a while, I had an entire week with no medical appointments – woo hoo!

My in-laws bought a new recliner, and gave us their old one. That became my new "feeding chair" in the den.

I had another esophagus dilation, but still couldn't swallow food. Sigh.

I had a recurring dream in which I was in a restaurant ordering food. Then I suddenly realized I couldn't eat the food I had ordered.

Meal planning was sometimes a challenge. I needed to feed 4 times a day, and it couldn't be done in public. There was no "grab and go" meal option for me; no "fast food". If I was going to be out for several hours, I had to really time it right to get all of my meals in.

Each year in September, we used to go to the Maryland Renaissance Festival. Although there are activities and shows to watch, the food was such a huge part of the experience that I could not go back this year.

Gratitude for the month:

Thankful for grandson on the way!

Food I miss this month – Scotch Eggs!

Children are the rainbow of life.
Grandchildren are the pot of gold.

Irish Blessing

<u>Chapter 11</u>
October
Weight: 125
Number of medical appointments: 3

There were several social food-type events this month.

First was the baby shower for my daughter-in-love. What a great time! Her stepmother and sister made all the arrangements. It was outdoors at a local park, and they had a fun "tie-dye a onesie for the baby" event, men included, and there were none of those gross shower games like "guess which candy bar has been smushed into this diaper?"! (*Shudder*) Possibly the best baby shower I'd ever attended.

We celebrated Rosh Hashanah with the in-laws. More food! But it was ok. Good to see everyone, and I tried to stay focused on the people and not the food I was missing. We decided to skip Yom Kippur, as it was just too much too soon.

My work holds an annual golf outing and reception, and I assist each year. At the reception, the servers come around with hors d'oeuvres. They kept coming at me with mini crab cakes and I kept saying "wish I could" or "none for me, thanks". Still easier to handle than a sit-down dinner. The room has several high top tables and a few seats, but most people walk around all evening and no one notices whether you are eating or not.

We went to a birthday party for a friend's grandson who turned 1. Food again, but what I missed out on more was the swimming pool! I love to swim, but with small kids around, I was afraid one of them would grab onto the tube right through my swimsuit - eeeekkk - so I didn't even try, just stuck my feet in.

Mid-month, I had to get the tube replaced again. Not an emergency this time, but the external tube was getting bent up and would not flush completely. After the tube was replaced each time, there was an adjustment period that was uncomfortable. It is hard to explain, but several times a day the tube would "suck in" and the disk would press into my stomach for several seconds at a time. Sometimes it would stop me in my tracks and I would have to put my hand over it until it "popped up" and released. This led to a hunched position, in which my upper body bent over protecting the tube area. My posture has never been great, but it was definitely worse during those times.

The biggest news came on the 27th, when my grandson entered the world! I visited the hospital the evening of his birth day. I greeted him the same way I greeted my granddaughter at first sight – "well hello, handsome (beautiful) genius!" As you know, all grandchildren are beautiful/ handsome geniuses! What a happy day!

On Halloween, I dressed up as Ferris Bueller at work. It was funny to hear all the variations of ways people mis-remembered his name. Then I tagged along when my son took my granddaughter trick or treating. So much fun watching her run from house to house. For a while she was going around with a candy bar sticking out of her mouth!

Gratitude for the month:

Thankful for my healthy grandson! My husband, sons, daughters-in-law, granddaughter. So blessed!

Food I miss this month – Arby's mozzarella sticks!

I am grateful for what I am and have.
My Thanksgiving is perpetual.

Henry David Thoreau

<u>Chapter 12</u>
November
Weight: 126
Number of medical appointments: 1

As this is the month for giving thanks, let's begin the chapter with gratitude instead of waiting until the end. I am grateful as always for my husband, sons, daughters-in-law, and grandchildren. I am grateful for all the things I CAN do – getting back to work full time, occasional grandchild babysitting, and helping Mom out with grocery shopping and banking. I am grateful for my secondary and tertiary families, that is, my in-laws and my coworkers, and of course my friends. I have all the support anyone could ever need from all of these wonderful people- truly blessed.

I had a "gratitude jar" in my kitchen. It was just a small labeled "Mason" jar with a pen and slips of paper nearby so we could jot down things we were grateful for as we stopped to notice them. We filled it up throughout the year, and emptied it and read over and re-appreciated everything at the New Year.

I went to a bridal shower for a friend's daughter this month – yup, I am THAT OLD – my friends' kids are getting married! Although I couldn't enjoy the food part of it, it was still fun. I've known this girl since she was about 4 years old, and I was glad to see her excited about marrying her man.

The presidential election this year was a tough one. For the first time, I was extremely unhappy with the country's choice. When I came in to work the following day, I stopped at a coworker's desk (who I happened to know voted against this candidate as I did) and we both started crying! I allowed myself one day to grieve over it, then it was time to move on and live with the decision, at least for the next four years.

I tried a different swallow and speech therapist, beginning this month. We ended up working more on my speech, and it helped. As for the swallowing, my doctor thinks there is just not enough tongue muscle left after several surgeries to move the food back to swallow. Before this adventure, I did not realize the swallowing process varied so much from liquids to solids.

My speech was impaired, but for the most part it was understandable. The most difficult sounds were the hard C and hard G, like in "cat" or "gate". If I reminded myself to speak more slowly, it worked better. If I was speaking to a stranger on the phone, I said "bear with me" before attempting a word that was harder to say – this helped, because it caused them to really listen. I don't see much karaoke in my future, but those who've heard me in years past would likely applaud that!

We celebrated Thanksgiving at my sister-in-law's house. Probably the most awkward holiday, because it is so food-centric. I tried instead to concentrate on connecting with family members that we don't see often. For example, we met our nephew's girlfriend for the first time. Also a longtime family friend and her family came from out of state.

This month saw my first time babysitting my grandson. He was still getting used to me, and seemed quite relieved to see his parents return home, but I loved every minute of it anyway.

Ok, more info for my peg tube brothers and sisters:
This month, the area around the tube got really itchy, like a diaper rash. I tried some over the counter ointments, but no go. My primary care doctor took a look, said it looked infected, gave me an antibiotic and it cleared up. However, weeks later it happened again. Back to the doctor - no antibiotic this time. A friend at work sells "Plexus" health products and gave me some samples of their Body Cream. So soothing! It looks weird because it is gray; it contains charcoal. It worked when nothing else would, so I bought a bottle. I have never bought any of their other products, but this one really worked for me so I figured I would give them a shout out. Another thing that helped was changing the gauze around the tube more frequently. Kind of a hassle, but better than being itchy!

November 30 marked one year since my oral cancer surgery. It had been quite a year, but I was thankful to be alive and healthy.

Food I miss this month – stuffing!

<u>**Afterword**</u>

I ended up keeping the feeding tube much longer than expected. I stopped using it in early June of the following year, having figured out how to get all my nutrition by mouth in liquid form. I had a follow up appointment in June with my gastro doc, and I was hoping to get the tube removed. He did not want to remove it yet, and though I was VERY disappointed, I agreed. Before my next appointment in September, I typed up a letter to convince him to remove it. I'm including a copy - in appendix 2 - in case any of you need an example for a similar experience. It worked! The tube was removed on September 26th – a happy day!

I can chew solid food, but can't swallow it. At least I can get an occasional taste of my favorites. I'm getting used to the liquid diet, a combination of Ensure and homemade smoothies with fruit and veggies added – recipes in appendix 3.

Here are 2 small things to be thankful for while on a liquid diet:

    1 – No more battle of the bulge – my weight has remained steady for years now.

    2 – I never have to wait in the "microwave line" at work (2 microwaves, 20 people eating lunch at once). I just grab my Ensure from the fridge, and lunch is ready!

Food events are easier to handle now. A few months after the tube removal, I finally invited my sons and their families over for dinner. I made dinner for everyone, and I sat at the table and drank my smoothie. I wasn't uncomfortable at all – of course being at home does make a difference. I was so happy to have all my favorite people in the house!

I've continued making the recovery kits mentioned in chapter 8. It's become a mission, and has expanded from illness/surgery recovery to new job kits and cheer up kits. One of my friends has joined in and we've made several kits together. Still paying it forward!

As of this writing, I have been cancer-free for over 4 years. I'm hopeful that going through the radiation treatments was the key to getting rid of it for good. My oral surgeon has extended my check-up intervals, so I only have to see him every 6 months - the longest interval I've had since I became his patient 20 years ago. The day we got news of the interval extension was another happy day!

Also, some happy family news – this past July, we were blessed with a second granddaughter!

Thank you for sharing in my journey, dear reader. I wish you good health and happiness.

There's a common denominator in our human experience. Everybody wants to know:
Did you hear me, and did what I say matter?
Oprah Winfrey

<u>**Acknowledgements/Love and Gratitude**</u>

Whew, where to start?...............
I'm feeling rebellious, so I will start where most acknowledgements end, with my family.

Thank you.
To my husband, Mike: Your love and support, both emotional and practical, carry me through all the dark days and make the good days even brighter.
To my sons, Scott and Chris, and my daughter-in-law Nicole: You are each amazing and wonderful in your own special way. Thank you for your encouragement and support.
To my beautiful genius grandchildren: Autumn, Lucas, and Audrey. You are the lights of my life, the apples of my eye, and the best motivation for me to stay healthy and stick around to watch you grow up and make this world a better place.
To my sisters, Lynne and June: If I needed an encouraging word, a break, a laugh, or a sounding board, you were there.
To my second family, my in-laws: Thank you for all you have done. I sure got lucky marrying into such a wonderful group of people.
To my third family, my bosses and coworkers at Acme Paper & Supply Company: Thank you for keeping me employed, and for your encouragement, support, and compassion. I am impressed daily by the fantastic group of people I am blessed to work with.
To all my doctors, nurses, and techs at the University of Maryland, especially Dr. Robert Ord and Martha Francis, NP: Your bedside manners are the best, and going through this process was easier with both of you in charge.
To my Facebook friends and family: Several times I shared that I was committed to working on the book every day for a month. I asked you to help hold me accountable to keep going, and you did!
To all my advance readers: the Maryland Writers' Association's first page panel, Mike, Scott, Chris, Lynne, Heather, Antony, Carol, Maggie, Vicky, Debra, and Cher. Your comments and suggestions made this a much better work.
Special thanks to Scott for all of the suggested corrections – I couldn't believe how many punctuation changes were needed! And to my cousin-by-marriage Antony – it meant so much to receive such encouraging feedback from a published author whose work I respect and enjoy.
It was very enlightening to hear some chapters read aloud – it is a good way to catch sentences that don't flow well. Thanks for recording them for me, Heather.
Heather also helped with formatting the eBook and selecting a cover. Extra thanks!
Lastly, I thank YOU, dear reader. Where would a book be without a reader, after all?

<u>**Appendix 1 (for my fellow tubies)**</u>

<u>*If you are new to the feeding tube experience, here is what we learned by trial and error:*</u>
Keep a towel handy when feeding, in case of spillover.

The feeding tube needs occasional replacing; I've heard 6-12 months.

Enteral nutrition products: Osmolite 1.5 caused bathroom issues, switched to Jevity 1.5 with fiber, no further problems. We used both Coram CVS Specialty Infusion Services and Byram Healthcare to order enteral nutrition.

Tube replacement can be messy; protect your clothes or ask for a gown. The process is fairly simple and quick. If your tube is like mine, they deflate the balloon through a small hole in the exterior part, remove the old tube and put the new one right in. Make sure the new tube is ready to insert before the doctor removes the old one. I got an infection twice after a delay in inserting the new tube; I'm not sure if it was related, BUT I did not get an infection after a different doctor replaced it quickly.

Gauze and tapes we used:

There is a type of gauze called a "drain sponge" with a split to accommodate the tube – we found McKesson brand to be reasonably priced and effective. As I mentioned in chapter 6, we ended up making the hole at the center larger so the gauze would not stick to the sensitive tissue.

We used paper tape to attach the gauze and to tape up the tube end so it did not dangle loosely. I have sensitive skin, and even the paper tape was irritating, but it was better than the other types. For showering, we used no gauze, and taped up the tube using Johnson and Johnson's Band-Aid brand waterproof tape to keep the tube out of the way.

Only upon researching for this book did I discover something called a "g-tube holder" – a washable elastic belt with a pouch that holds the tubing close to the body. This seems like a winner, and would have saved us a LOT of money on tape. We kept hoping that I wouldn't have the tube very long; I guess that is why we never took the time to research and learn about products like this.

I discovered this online support group later, when doing some research - check it out, it may help you: https://www.inspire.com/groups/oley-foundation/

Keeping your focus on gratitude is always helpful. Find something to be thankful for each day. You don't even have to write it down -though it is fun to re-read later - just notice and feel the gratitude in the moment.

Looking for good news? Try these (I follow both on Facebook):
https://www.goodgoodgood.co/goodnewspaper
https://tanksgoodnews.com/

If you prefer email newsletters, this is a good one, and it is weekly – I prefer that over the daily ones:
https://www.cnn.com/specials/us/the-good-stuff

Prescription mouth rinse: Caphosol – very beneficial when dealing with radiation side effects. This is an expensive one – if your insurance won't cover it, appeal to them and to your doctors/hospital for assistance.

Books: Laughter Therapy by Ace McCloud, Kid President's Guide to Being Awesome by Brad Montague and Robby Novak, Unlocking the Heart of Healing by Bridget Hughes, Complete Tubefeeding by Eric Adhaar O'Gorman

Plexus Body Cream https://plexusworldwide.com/product/plexus-body-cream
This is the cream that helped heal the itchiness around the tube incision.

Barbara Hauf Cancer Foundation
This organization provides grants to cancer patients who have worked in the lawn and garden industry.

Greenpath debt management -
http://www.greenpath.com/how-we-can-help/debt-management-plan
This company helped me get on track with my credit card debt.

Strawberry or Vanilla Ensure Enlive -
My favorite of all the nutrition drinks – 350 calories per serving, the highest calorie count I've seen on this type of drink. It contains 20 grams protein and 3 grams dietary fiber. It does have 20 grams of sugar, which is worth noting. I drink one of these for lunch each day.

Suction machine – this was necessary after surgery when I could not swallow. Fortunately, my insurance covered it 100% and we had it at our home for months.

Fluoride gel for trays – I used Gel-Kam first but it yellowed my teeth – switched to Prevident, much better. Also it comes in Very Berry flavor! Mint burns my mouth. I have to use the fluoride trays once a day forever, due to the radiation treatment. In addition, I use an extra-fluoride prescription toothpaste, also by Prevident. Their non-mint flavor is called Fruitastic.

<u>**Appendix 2 - Letter to my gastro doc – arguments for tube removal:**</u>

<u>Why I no longer need the tube:</u>
- I have not used the tube for 3 months. I get all my nutrition by mouth. I use a combination of Ensure drinks and Carnation breakfast essentials mixed with coconut and almond milks, nut butters, fruit, vegetables, and a fiber supplement. I will be adding some blended soups to the mix as well, and will continue to try different foods and improve my nutrition further.

- As to the risk of having a sore throat and being unable to swallow – my throat was quite sore after the last esophagus dilation, but I was still able to get all my liquid meals down.

<u>Things I am able to do without using the tube:</u>
- Maintain my health and weight with a liquid diet
- Work full time, including a fairly long commute
- Babysit my 2 active grandchildren
- Assist in caring for my elderly mother and her home

<u>Why I no longer want the tube:</u>
- It contributes to my sense of "other". Bad enough I have scars, can't eat solids, and have speech impairment – I also have this appendage sticking out of my stomach. I feel like I am done with cancer, so I don't want this "accessory" any longer, as a reminder of the experience.

- The skin around the tube gets itchy. Also, even the gentle paper tape irritates my fair, unreasonably sensitive skin.

- I have to deal with it 3 times a day; 2 bandage changes and using waterproof tape for the shower.

- The unused tube is gross – though I'm not putting anything in, stomach contents still come out into the external tube.

The bottom line: I want the tube removed. I am willing to take any risk you feel is involved.

<u>**Appendix 3 - recipes:**</u>

<u>Homemade mouth rinse</u> - I started using this after radiation treatments and still use it once a day:

2 cups warm water
1 teaspoon salt
1 teaspoon baking soda
Mix and store. Swish approximately 1 tablespoon of the rinse for 30 seconds each morning and rinse with water.
I found a pretty, small "cruet" type jar with a cork (at Michaels craft store) – I use this to store my mouth rinse – it reminds me of something from Harry Potter.

<u>Typical breakfast smoothie:</u>

½ cup almond milk
½ cup coconut milk (I use Trader Joe's reduced fat; it has more calories and less sugar than some others)
½ cup fruit pieces (I prefer a combination of apple and banana, and sometimes mango)
spinach leaves
red bell pepper pieces
Occasional frozen veggie substitutions: green beans, sliced carrots, butternut squash cubes
canned pumpkin (2 tablespoons – I freeze the pumpkin in an ice cube tray)
Carnation breakfast essentials – 1 packet
1 serving NutriSource fiber supplement (flavorless, effective, dissolves well)
½ Flintstones multivitamin
1 tablespoon peanut butter (we make this at home, more on that later)
1 tablespoon sunflower seed butter

I use a NutriBullet blender, but a standard blender works too. Occasionally I add a little treat, like a cut-up s'mores Girl Scout cookie!
Blend, strain if needed, add ice.

<u>Homemade peanut butter:</u>

You need a sturdy blender for this. We have a Blendtec that came with a special jar and blade specifically for making nut butters. We buy dry roasted unsalted peanuts, and that is the ONLY INGREDIENT. It has to be refrigerated, and would be a bit runny for sandwiches, but it is perfect for smoothies - and we like the fact that neither salt nor thickeners are added. We store it in Rubbermaid glass containers.

<u>Typical dinner smoothie</u>:

½ cup almond milk
½ cup coconut milk
½ cup fruit pieces
spinach leaves
red bell pepper pieces
Occasional frozen veggie substitutions: green beans, sliced carrots, butternut squash cubes
Carnation breakfast essentials light start (less sugar) – 1 packet
½ Flintstones multivitamin
1 tablespoon peanut butter
1 tablespoon cashew butter (Trader Joe's)
Blend, strain if needed, add ice.

<u>4thmeal smoothie</u>:
½ cup almond milk
½ cup coconut milk
Carnation breakfast essentials light start – 1 packet
1 tablespoon peanut butter
1 tablespoon mixed nut butter (Trader Joe's)

Blend, strain if needed, add ice.

Note – to get all my calories in for the day, I consume 4 meals, including an Ensure at lunch time. If you can fit all of your daily calories into 3 meals, your meal prep schedule will be much more manageable.

<u>**Appendix 4 – medical details:**</u>

Type of cancer:
Moderately differentiated squamous cell carcinoma on right tongue. I am a bit of an anomaly among my doctor's many patients, as my first incidence was on my left tongue, and since then everything has been on the right side - most patients have recurrences always on the same side.

Surgery:
Once the cancer was removed from my tongue, the tissue had to be replaced. This was done with a "forearm flap" which is a living graft, including blood vessels, taken from my forearm and attached in my mouth. Then a skin graft was taken from my leg to replace the skin on my forearm.

Scars, from this and previous surgeries:
3 white patches on left thigh – all skin graft donor sites – largest is about 2 x 4 inches.
Rectangular area on left forearm - living donor site, with a white line going up toward elbow
½ inch long vertical scar below lower lip
L shaped scar on right neck
Small scar at base of neck from tracheostomy tube
"2nd belly button" on left side of abdomen from feeding tube

My favorite quote regarding scars:

Never be ashamed of a scar. It simply means you were stronger than whatever tried to hurt you.
(The author is unknown.)

<u>**About the Author**</u>

Robin Hommel is a wife, mom, grandma, office worker, proofreader, writer, and artist. This is her first book. She lives in Maryland with her awesome husband, lots of books, and a couple of decent houseplants.